Acid Reflux Diet

Your Guide To Eating Right For Your Body And Curing Your Symptoms Today!

Book Description

Acid reflux is not a pleasant thing to have to live with. The irritation, the pain, and being unable to enjoy a variety of foods makes it difficult for you to be able to enjoy eating out with friends and family, and may even make it difficult to get out of bed and enjoy going to work or getting through your day.

With acid reflux, you never know what is going to trigger your symptoms, or what is going to cause you to fall into a bout of discomfort and make doing anything a real challenge. In spite of all the pills, remedies, and various things your doctor tells you to do, you know better than anyone that life with acid reflux is difficult.

If only there was a way for you to help your symptoms without having to turn to synthetic pills. If only there was a way for you to live without fear of a flare up, or without wondering if your acid reflux is going to kick in and ruin your day. If only there was a way for you to handle your acid reflux symptoms through your lifestyle rather than through medication.

That's where this book comes in. In it, you are going to learn everything you need to know to manage your acid reflux symptoms through diet and exercise alone. There is no need for you to take those synthetic pills, and there's no need for you to live in worry that you are going to get sick at a bad time.

With the acid reflux diet, you live in a way that allows you to live fully, without fear that your acid reflux is going to flare up and leave you lying in bed in a world of pain. With the remedies outlined in this book, you're going to take control of your life back, and live life to the fullest.

- **Learn how to manage your acid reflux through your lifestyle choices**

- **Learn the options you have with your acid reflux and how to minimize flare ups**

- **Learn how to enjoy life without having to constantly worry about your acid reflux**

- **And much, much more!**

Table of Contents

Introduction

You love pizza. And spaghetti. And breakfast foods, and citrus fruit. You love pineapple and oranges, lemonade and tomato juice. You could live happily if you only ever got to eat Italian foods for the rest of your life. Yes, you love the spices and the sauces, the fresh twist of citrus, and everything that goes with it.

But you don't love flare ups. In fact, one of the worst things you can imagine is when that burning begins in your stomach and rushes up your esophagus. You want nothing more than cool relief, but you are only met with more and more pain.

You begin to wonder how you are going to spend the rest of your life like this. As you know, there is no cure for acid reflux, so you are left with the feeling that you are going to have to simply suck up the pain and live like this – regardless of how it is making you feel.

As someone who suffers from acid reflux, the thought of this is not a pleasant one. All you want is some relief – you want to be able to enjoy life with your friends and family and not have to deal with these annoying flare ups, or worry that you are going to get sick at any random moment.

You want to be able to go out to restaurants, and be able to enjoy barbecues and other family gatherings. You want to be able to enjoy a fresh glass of lemonade without worrying that it's going to set you back for days or even weeks.

If this describes you, then you have come to the right place. Imagine living a life in which you didn't have to worry about whether you were going to feel sick or not. Imagine what it would be like for you to get to enjoy yourself, knowing that you were controlling your symptoms through your lifestyle.

With the right guidance, this can be you, and I am going to show you how. I know how hard it can be living with acid reflux, and I know how much you appreciate the good days – especially after dealing with the bad. I want to give you the gift of living the good days, and never having to worry that you are going to experience those flare ups.

Let me show you the secret to controlling your acid reflux through your diet and lifestyle choices, and give you the gift of controlling this problem without having to give up on the things you love. With the right attitude and the right skills, you really can live life without having to take all those synthetic pills.

Acid reflux can be controlled and virtually eliminated through your lifestyle choices alone, so rest assured there is hope for you. This book is going to show you the secret you have been looking for.

Your best life awaits.

Chapter 1 –
What is Acid Reflux?

Acid reflux is one of the most misdiagnosed diseases there is. This is because many people will mistake the symptoms for something else, and not realize what is happening to their bodies.

Gastroesophageal reflux disease – which is more commonly referred to merely as acid reflux, can display itself in a variety of ways. The most common symptom of the disease is heartburn, which is often the only symptom people watch for when they suspect they have the disease.

In a healthy individual, there is a ring of muscle that opens and closes in the lower part of the esophagus. It is closed most of the time, and only opens when food is entering the stomach. This keeps all the acid in the stomach safely in the stomach where it belongs, and away from the sensitive esophagus area.

When an individual develops gastroesophageal reflux disease, this ring doesn't work properly, which allows the acid from the stomach to creep up and into the esophagus. This is what results in all the burning and painful sensations you feel in your throat and chest – why many people refer to it as heartburn.

Normal heartburn only lasts for a short period of time, and it doesn't come back. If you find that you are experiencing prolonged heartburn and that it comes back often, you should seek medical attention, as acid reflux that goes untreated will often result in further complications – but we will look more at that later.

Since acid reflux can cause many different complications, it's important to know what the other common symptoms are. As you know, this is one of the most misdiagnosed diseases there is, so many people live with it for years without ever knowing that they have it.

In addition to heartburn, other symptoms include:

•**Bloating** – bloating can be caused by a number of different conditions, but it is often associated with acid reflux. If you feel bloated often, get checked by a medical professional as soon as possible.

•**Burping** – unexplained burping, painful burping, or burping that tastes bad are all signs of stomach acid being in the esophagus.

•**Dark stool** – your bowel movements say a lot about your health. Dark stool often indicates that there is some sort of problem going on with the digestive tract, if you are experiencing this at any time consider going in to get checked by a professional.

•**Dysphagia** – difficulty swallowing will often indicate some sort of medical condition, it's wise to get it checked out if you are experiencing this symptom.

•**Nausea**

•**Unexplained weight loss**

•**Unexplained or prolonged sore throat (or a sore throat that keeps coming back)** – cold and flu season is one thing, but if you find that you have a sore throat – no matter how mild – that keeps coming back, go in and get it looked at.

•**Tasting stomach acid** – this is one of the prime indications that there is stomach acid in the esophagus.

•**Pain when you are lying down** – lying down makes it even easier for your stomach acid to creep into your esophagus, especially when your sphincter isn't working.

Whenever there is any change in your health or comfort, it's a good idea to get it looked at by a medical professional. There are many different conditions that can contribute to these symptoms, but keep in mind that acid reflux could be the culprit.

If you are going to the doctor for any of these symptoms, bring up acid reflux if your physician does not.

What causes acid reflux?

Although acid reflux is an incredibly common condition that affections millions of people around the globe, doctors and scientists are still learning about it. While there are certainly a lot of things we do know, there are still things that haven't been entirely confirmed.

Although there hasn't been any concrete evidence to confirm the actual cause of acid reflux, there are certain things that many doctors believe to be major contributing factors.

These are:

- **Living a poor lifestyle** – slouching when you stand or sit down, drinking, smoking, and being overweight all tend to be tied to acid reflux, as well as not taking care of one's health as they should.

- **Certain medical or physical conditions** – gaining weight too fast, pregnancy, hiatal hernia, diabetes, and certain other conditions appear to be a cause of acid reflux.

- **The way you consume your food** – eating too close to lying down (whether that be going to bed, taking a nap, or merely lying down after you eat a meal,) eating meals that are too large for your stomach to handle, and eating meals too quickly can cause this condition.

•Having a diet that is rich in spicy or hot foods – a diet that is rich in foods such as garlic, onions, spices (especially the hotter spices such as peppers and turmeric) or eating a lot of hot peppers themselves can be a leading factor that causes acid reflux.

•Certain medications – nitrates, antihistamines, and certain blood medications may be tied to acid reflux.

As you read through the list of symptoms and causes, you may see a correlation between how you live your life and the symptoms you are experiencing. If you suspect that you have acid reflux, it is incredibly important that you go to your doctor right away for a medical diagnosis.

Although many people would rather not know when there is something wrong with them, certain conditions must be taken care of if you wish to see relief from the symptoms you are feeling, and you want to go back to living life as you were before. Of course, to eliminate some of these symptoms you're going to have to make some big changes – but with the proper lifestyle you will be able to control how often you have a flare up.

Can acid reflux be cured?

Often a diagnosis of any kind will scare a person into going online and searching their symptoms to see if there might be some way they can be cured. They may or may not do this before seeing a doctor, but more often than not a person who has been diagnosed with a disease (or a person who suspects that they have a disease) will take to the internet in hopes of some answers.

If you were to search whether you can cure your acid reflux or not, you're going to run into mixed answers. There are those who are confident that you can cure the disease and go back to a life that is acid reflux free, then there are those who are certain that there is no cure for the disease and that you must live a life of management.

Of course, when you go to the doctor for your acid reflux, it is likely you will be given some kind of medication to help manage the symptoms – but medication isn't a cure. Whether you can cure your acid reflux through your diet and lifestyle choices may be unclear, but what is clear is that you can minimize and eliminate many of your symptoms through your lifestyle – which is something medication can't do.

When you use lifestyle choices for your health, you need to have the right mindset. If you are only going to make changes to cure an illness, it's likely you are going to stop when you see the symptoms go away – only to go back to your old habits and have your symptoms return.

When it comes to your health, you need to establish a healthy lifestyle that will keep you feeling your best regardless of symptoms you may have experienced in the past. With the acid reflux diet, you are going to make the changes your body needs to feel great day after day, but it's important that you stick with these changes even after you see your symptoms disappear.

As you have seen there are a lot of different causes for acid reflux, and in order to keep any of the symptoms from coming back, you're going to have to make changes in each of the areas you have seen. From taking care of yourself to how you eat to how you stand all plays a role in the symptoms of this disease.

Whether it can be cured or not is not the question – the question is: what will you do to ensure you never experience these symptoms again?

Chapter 2 –
Return of the Reflux: Side Effects

If you have been struggling with the symptoms of acid reflux, you will, no doubt, want some kind of relief from what you are feeling. There are those who get the symptoms hard, then there are those who have milder cases, but regardless of the extent of your symptoms, it's important that you do not ignore the condition.

It's a wonder how many people ignore their declining health, and continue to go through their lives living as they have always lived – even when that means they are suffering. However, as with other illnesses and diseases, ignored acid reflux can lead to some conditions that are much worse.

You can alleviate the symptoms with medication, but if you want to better your health and ensure you aren't going to develop anything worse, you're going to need to make some lifestyle changes.

Many people with acid reflux will eat what they want then take a pill afterward to ward off the burning and stinging, but this only stops the burning and stinging, it doesn't do anything for halting or reversing the condition.

Without making deliberate lifestyle changes, untreated acid reflux can lead to:

•**Esophageal Ulcers** – The stomach acid that creeps into the esophagus can eat away at the soft tissue lining the throat and result in painful ulcers.

•**Esophagitis** – Inflammation of the esophagus.

•**Buildup of scar tissue in the Esophagus** – As the stomach acid erodes away the layers of tissue surrounding the esophagus, it will be replaced with scar tissue that can build up over time.

•**Barret's Esophagus** – A condition in which unusual precancerous cells build up in the walls of the esophagus.

•**Increased risk of Esophageal Cancer** – Where there are precancer cells, there is a heightened risk of developing actual cancer – as you know this is going to lead to a host of other medical problems.

•**Tooth decay** – Stomach acid is very hard on the teeth and can erode the soft enamel, resulting in cavities, broken teeth, and root canals.

As you read through this list of potential medical problems that result from untreated acid reflux, you can see what a serious condition this really is. Although you may only be experiencing mild effects of the disease right now, you can see

11

that those symptoms aren't going to stay mild, and can turn into potentially deadly conditions.

Though medication will make you feel better at the time, it's not going to stop any of these other conditions from taking root unless you make some simple – yet serious – lifestyle changes. Don't worry, though it may seem like your life is going to drastically change right now, I am going to show you how easy it really is to gain your health back.

All you need is to know a few simple tips and tricks that will change your life immensely. Remember that practice makes perfect, and the only way for this to work in your life is if you are to stick with it in the long term. You can't stop when you see the symptoms starting to go away, and you can't stop when you think they have gone away completely.

If you have acid reflux now, you are going to be at risk for developing the symptoms again at any time – it's up to you to make sure that doesn't happen, and I'm going to show you how.

Chapter 3 –
You Are What You Eat: How Diets Control and Contribute to Acid Reflux

The saying *you are what you eat* has been around for hundreds of years, and though it has taken more of a cliché tone these days, truer words have never been spoken. Study after study has backed the fact that people who eat certain kinds of foods as a habit of life are going to have the health that goes with that diet.

For example:

It's no surprise to anyone that someone who lives off of fast food and a sedentary lifestyle is going to be overweight and unhealthy.

At the same time, it's no surprise that a person who makes a habit of eating healthy foods and taking care of his body is going to be a healthy weight with few health problems.

Body builders eat a lot of protein to ensure they build large muscles, while runners opt for a high carb diet to ensure they have the energy they need to make it through their runs.

Basically, if you were to look at a diet plan at any given time without being told who the plan was for, you would likely be able to pinpoint the kind of person who would eat that way – whether they are a health–conscious person, someone who is trying to lose weight, someone who is trying to gain weight, or someone who is trying to achieve some level of performance from their body through their diet.

When it comes to acid reflux, you are going to live life more like an athlete. Unlike those who go on diets to lose weight, you aren't going to avoid foods because you are worried about calories or that they are going to affect your body as far as fat goes, you are going to instead eat food based on your triggers.

As you know, there are certain foods that make your heartburn worse than others. This is likely what caused you to examine whether you had acid reflux in the first place.

Now, you may have this list of foods in the back of your mind that you can't eat because of your heartburn, but instead of looking at the list as a list of food names, I want to challenge you to look at the list of foods and find what they have in common.

For example:

Do you find that whenever you eat greasy foods you tend to get heartburn? Is it caffeine that makes your chest feel like it's on fire? Or is it fizzy drinks or soda that make you feel like your throat is in flames?

Are you one of those people who "can't eat Mexican or Italian?"

Take an honest look at your diet, and think about the foods that make you feel bad – connect the dots in your mind and determine what it is about these foods that make them alike, and you'll start to form a list of "triggers."

As we have already seen, at its core acid reflux occurs when the muscle at the bottom of your esophagus and above your stomach doesn't close properly, which allows the stomach acid to creep out of your stomach and into your esophagus. Though it is unclear why certain foods make this happen in certain people while other foods do not, it's important to know which of those foods cause this to happen in you.

When it comes to acid reflux, there is no universal rule that works for every person every time – it comes down to what works for *you* and when. There are those with acid reflux who have no problem drinking tea or coffee, then there are those with the same condition who can't have any coffee or they find that their throat is on fire.

Some people do fine with things like garlic and onions, while others do not. If you haven't been keeping track of what your triggers are, then grab a notebook and a pen, and track what you are eating for a couple weeks. Write down the foods that cause you to flare up and look for a pattern.

This may be a specific food (for example, coffee gives you heartburn) or it might be a little subtler (garlic bread gives you heartburn, garlic mushrooms give you heartburn, that garlicy soup from your favorite restaurant gives you heartburn – garlic is the common denominator.)

Learn what your own personal triggers are, and you'll be much better able to avoid the foods that cause it to happen.

While it's incredibly important to know what causes your acid reflux to flare up, that's only half the battle. The other half is learning what soothes your symptoms or keeps them at bay altogether.

Acid reflux is a two-way street. Though you are going to spend time focusing on what causes it and avoiding those, it's also important to know what can alleviate your symptoms. Like putting together the pieces of a puzzle, you're going to learn how to live not only to avoid symptoms, but to actively soothe them.

Our bodies are designed to respond to the foods and substances we put inside ourselves. Your body is going to use the food you eat in as many ways as it can, whether that be in a way that aggravates your symptoms, or a way that heals itself.

Listen to your body, and do what you can to give it what it needs to get rid of your acid reflux. Though I will provide you with a list of foods that are common triggers as well as a list of foods that usually help, there is going to be a time of trial and error on your part.

Learn what works for you in your situation, and begin conquering your symptoms today.

Chapter 4 –
The Spice of Life: Dietary Do's and Don'ts for Acid Reflux

In the last chapter, you saw how diets can directly contribute to your acid reflux condition, whether that contribution is in a good way or a bad way. You also learned that you need to discover what it is in your life personally that contributes to your condition and how you can control your symptoms through your lifestyle choices.

While it is true that no two people are alike, and something that works for you may or may not work for another, there do tend to be common triggers (and soothers) for those who are struggling with this disease. With this in mind, we are going to look at what those foods are on both ends of the spectrum, and give you a head start for your own dietary needs.

First, let's look at the list of foods that are commonly known to cause acid reflux symptoms:

•**Alcohol** – red wine and beer appear to be the worst for causing acid reflux symptoms, although all alcohol can be a culprit. Alcohol relaxes your body (which will, in turn, relax the sphincter to your stomach) and can potentially cause acid to creep back into your esophagus.

•**Fried foods/fast foods** – avoid foods that have been fried in any way, even if you are cooking at home. Excess oil tends to aggravate symptoms.

•**Spicy foods** – hot spices are the worse – turmeric, peppers, foods that have been cooked to be "hot."

•**Tomatoes** – this is due to the acid content.

•**Oranges** – again, this is due to the acid content.

•**Mint** – mint relaxes the esophagus and can cause acid to come in.

•**Beef** – though you will find many acid reflux recipes with this ingredient, it's important to note that it's not all beef that causes triggers. Avoid beef that is high in fat, and always opt for the lean varieties.

•**Coffee** – caffeine tends to be a trigger for many people, although there are those who don't experience the same effects. If you are going to drink coffee or tea, go for the decaffeinated varieties.

•**Cheese** – again because of the fat content. When you select cheese, go for the low fat or fat free varieties.

•**Soda** – carbonation can cause a buildup of gas in the stomach, and thus put pressure on the sphincter. If soda is a problem for you, avoid all carbonated beverages.

•**Chocolate** – chocolate has caffeine, it's potentially high in fat, and it has sugar in it. All three of these can cause acid reflux symptoms.

•**Garlic** – certain spice levels in this ingredient will aggravate symptoms for acid reflux in some people.

•**Onions** – certain spice levels in this ingredient will aggravate symptoms for acid reflux in some people.

•**Salt and peppers** – certain spice levels in these ingredients will aggravate symptoms for acid reflux in some people.

•**Butter** – look out for the fat content. If you are going to use butter, consider going with a non–dairy alternative.

•**Candy** – sugar has been known to cause symptoms in some people. Listen to your body.

•**Milk** – again look out for the fat content. Many people who have problems with milk find that low fat and fat free varieties don't cause symptoms.

When you first read over the list, it can feel a bit overwhelming – it seems that many of the foods you normally eat appear, which makes you wonder what there will be for you to enjoy in your cooking. However, if you notice the reason many of these foods cause symptoms to flare up, you can opt for other varieties of the same foods to get what you enjoy.

If you like beef, use lean varieties. Avoid the skin of chickens, as this is where the most fat is found. Enjoy fat free or low fat dairy products, and avoid caffeine. For all the foods on the list, there are many options out there that you can try.

We must not forget, avoiding certain foods is only half the battle. Let's look at a list of foods now that help keep the acid reflux symptoms at bay in most people.

•**Green leafy vegetables**

•**Ginger**

•**Oatmeal**

•**Lean meats**

•**Non–citrus fruits**

•**Egg whites**

•**Healthy fats**

That's right. Not only will avoiding fatty meats help with the triggering of your symptoms, but the addition of lean meats can potentially help keep your symptoms at bay.

In addition, you know you are going to avoid fats found in most products, but at the same time you need to try to bring in healthy fats. Avocados, nuts, flax seeds, etc. are all loaded with healthy fats that will keep your symptoms from coming back.

When it comes to acid reflux and your body, the only thing you can really do is pay attention to your health and listen to what your body is telling you. There may be things on the trigger list that don't both you, and there may be things on the list of good foods that do.

Therefore, it is incredibly important for you to keep a food journal – this way you will know without a doubt the ingredients you can use, the ingredients you should use, and the ingredients you need to avoid at all cost.

But, you may be wondering, what is it in these foods that causes flare ups? What is it you need to be keeping an eye on when it comes to your diet and eating plan?

As with all science, there is a reason behind the phenomenon that happens, and in the next chapter, I am going to show you what you need to be paying attention to. A healthy lifestyle (and an acid reflux diet) goes beyond just a list of healthy foods versus a list of foods that are unhealthy.

Read on to discover the why behind the method, and equip yourself with the knowledge you need to make your own choices in the diet realm.

Chapter 5 –
The PH Battle

You remember sitting in science class and listening to your teacher discuss alkaline and PH levels. You learned that one end of the scale was basic and the other end of the scale as acidic – with a fair number of experiments to go along with them.

The human body can also be found on the PH scale in several ways. Each part of your body is on the scale in a different place, with your stomach being on the acidic side of the scale and your blood being on the alkaline side of the scale – with your other organs and members being found all across the board.

It may come as a surprise to you to learn that when you are struggling with acid reflux, you are actually dealing with a low amount of acid in your stomach. Many people assume that you get reflux when you have too much acid in your stomach and it creeps through the sphincter, but this isn't always the case.

Your stomach is supposed to be the holding compartment for stomach acid. It's where the acid is created, it's where the acid should be stored, and it's where the food is largely broken down before it finishes its digestive journey.

When you are dealing with acid reflux, the acid that is created in your stomach creeps into your esophagus, resulting in a lower amount of stomach acid. It's no surprise that your body is a system that works with itself in a variety of ways, and when one part of that system is out of balance, the other parts of the body aren't going to work as they should, either.

The food you eat affects your body in a variety of ways – many of the foods found on the list of triggers are foods that cause your body to become more acidic as a whole – something you don't want for your acid reflux.

The goal of the acid reflux diet is to eat foods that don't cause your condition to become worse, and to incorporate foods which cause your body to balance. As you shop, cook, and eat look for foods that give your body the desired effect you wish to achieve.

There are dozens of online resources with lists of foods and where they fall on the PH scale. Look into those and base your shopping and cooking on the PH levels of the food you choose to eat. Talk to your doctor about what is recommended for your acid reflux, and ask about which foods you should try to incorporate into your diet on a daily basis.

Don't be afraid to make a list of the foods and the way they affect your body with their PH levels, then get your doctor's opinion on which you should stay away from, and which you should choose. As I have said before, your body is going to react in the way that it does that is entirely unique to you. Though there are very specific charts and things you can look at that will help with your decisions, you must remember that there is also trial and error involved.

Work with your body to find what works for you, and opt for foods that make you feel your best. This could be the same list as other people you know, or you may include foods that only you are able to eat with your acid reflux. The end goal is to make sure you aren't experiencing acid reflux symptoms. However you can make that happen with the foods you are eating, go with that.

The human body is designed much like a machine. The food you put into your body is the fuel your body needs to function properly.

Too many people settle into the typical diet of fast food and convenience, without ever truly considering the long–term effect such things have on the body. When they become ill with any kind of disease, they immediately turn to using medications to manage the symptoms, though they don't do a thing to change their lifestyles.

The more you can learn about the food you are putting into your body and the things that food does to your body, the better off you will be making decisions for your health.

It does take time, and it takes an immense amount of effort, but in the end, it's worth it. You can't put a price on your health, and though it can be confusing and even frustrating to work with your body until you are able to get it under control, it's worth it.

Get online now, and search for lists of the PH of the common foods you eat, and what those foods do to your body. Search for the kinds of foods that are going to work with your body and alleviate the acid reflux symptoms, then focus on cooking with those foods exclusively.

At the end of this book you are going to find a few recipes that will get you started on the right path with your acid reflux and lay the foundation for your cooking in the future.

Chapter 6 –
Immediate Relief: Remedies for Sudden Symptoms

As you have seen time and time again throughout this book, acid reflux is a disease. All those painful things you are feeling are the symptoms that indicate that you have this disease – they aren't the disease itself. You see, if you were to consider the base issue you are dealing with when you have acid reflux, you would see that the problem is with the muscle at the top of your stomach and the base of your esophagus.

At its most basic form, your problem is that this muscle isn't working properly, and as a result you are experiencing a variety of adverse side effects – the heartburn, the difficulty sleeping and swallowing, and everything else that goes along with this disease.

Throughout this book, I have been showing you a variety of ways you can alleviate the symptoms you are feeling, and help you get over this reflux. However, as with all other diseases, there is always a chance that you are going to experience sudden symptoms without warning. When this happens, you are going to want immediate relief – even without medication.

There's nothing wrong with having acid reflux medication on hand for your symptoms or to

help treat the disease itself, although you are going to primarily be treating it through your diet and lifestyle choices.

However, there are also a variety of natural things you can do that will alleviate the symptoms you are feeling, and many of them work as well if not better than the medications.

Here is a list of things you can do when you feel that familiar flare up – try them out and find the ones that work the best, then keep them on hand for when you have those sudden attacks.

Fast relief will be on the way:

> •**Teaspoon of baking soda** – whenever you feel an acid reflux attack coming on, or if you wake up and you are already feeling the effects of the burn, mix 1 teaspoon of baking soda with ½ cup warm water and drink it quickly.

The baking soda will help neutralize the acid in your throat and provide that much–needed relief as quickly as possible.

> •**Tablespoon of aloe juice** – just as with the baking soda, you can follow the same recipe to bring relief with aloe juice. Mix 1 tablespoon of the aloe juice with ½ cup of warm water and drink it quickly.

Though it is true you want to watch how quickly you consume your food to avoid the attack in the first place, if you are enduring the symptoms of an attack you want to bring relief to your body as quickly as possible. With this in mind, drink up.

> •**Proper posture** – if you are having an attack, keep your chin pointed toward the sky and don't lie down. Your goal is to keep the stomach in the right position as much as possible, and help your body heal.

> •**Chew gum** – you can use minty flavors if you like, or go with another flavor – both have been shown to help with an acid reflux attack.

> •**Take apple cider vinegar** – although it sounds counterproductive, drinking apple cider vinegar will actually help your body return to its normal PH levels, and make you feel better. If you are enduring an attack, mix 1 tablespoon of ACV with 1 glass of water and drink quickly.

To use ACV to prevent further attacks, you are going to mix 1 tablespoon of ACV with 1 glass of water and enjoy it 3 times per day. It doesn't matter what times you drink it, you just need to spread it out throughout the day.

> •**Drink ginger tea** – ginger has been known to help with stomach problems for thousands

of years, and acid reflux is no exception. If you feel an attack coming on, or if you wake up and are already feeling the burn, brew a glass of ginger tea and drink it as quickly as you can.

You will begin feeling relief within minutes of finishing.

•Chew on ginger root – again, ginger has been known to help with stomach problems for thousands of years, and acid reflux is no exception. If you feel an attack coming on, or if you wake up and are already feeling the burn, chew on crystalized ginger root or just a thin slice of ginger until you feel the symptoms start to subside.

You will begin feeling relief within minutes of finishing.

•Try mustard – as with the apple cider vinegar, few people think that mustard would help when you are feeling an acid reflux attack. But, as with the apple cider vinegar, mustard helps your body return to its normal balance.

You can use mustard throughout your day or you can try a teaspoon of it if you are in the middle of an attack. If you choose to spread it on something make sure that you go basic with the item so you don't put your body into overdrive with more acid.

31

•**Drink chamomile tea** – if you are looking for a sweeter tea to alleviate your symptoms rather than ginger, go with chamomile. Known for its ability to soothe the stomach, chamomile will help with both your stomach and your throat when you are enduring an acid reflux attack. Brew a cup of this warm liquid when you feel an attack coming on and drink it quickly, or brew it during the heartburn and sip on it.

Either way you are going to feel immediate relief rushing through your entire body.

•**Eat a handful of almonds** – we have long known that almonds are good for the body in a variety of ways, but few people realize that they will actually help with the symptoms you feel from your acid reflux.

As with some of these other remedies, you can eat them during the attack for relief, or you can eat them throughout the day to help ward off an attack in the first place. Opt for the plain, unsalted, uncoated varieties to keep from aggravating your symptoms in another way.

•**Eat a red delicious apple** – this is an excellent preventative method as well as a remedy for when acid reflux strikes. You can slice up a red delicious apple and enjoy it after a meal to help prevent any of the symptoms from showing up in the first place, or you can slice one and enjoy it when you are in the middle of an attack.

It is important to note that you must eat the red delicious apple, as other apples don't tend to offer the same results, nor is there a way to know what kind of apples are used with the apple juice you have in your cupboard. Stock up on these apples, and keep them on hand for when you are having an attack.

•Drink a cup of warm water mixed with lemon juice – although you want to avoid lemons most of the time to prevent an attack from happening in the first place, certain studies have shown that if you drink warm lemon water when you are experiencing heartburn it does offer some relief.

Keep a bottle of organic lemon juice on hand for when you are experiencing these attacks, and you'll find relief faster than you ever thought possible.

When it comes to the world of natural remedies and treating disease and illness through your lifestyle, it is always better to opt for prevention rather than remedies. Everything you can do to stop an outbreak from happening in the first place is going to work a lot easier than if you were to live like you have been living and are looking for ways to alleviate the symptoms you feel.

However, even with the best care there is still a chance that you may end up experiencing symptoms from time to time, and at that point it doesn't matter how hard you worked to prevent them – you are still feeling them at the moment.

With this in mind, it's important that you know what you can use to offer immediate relief. No one enjoys experiencing the symptoms, and many people are hit hard enough that they are bedridden even though the last thing they want to do is be in their beds.

Acid reflux is a complex disease and needs to be treated in both ways – do what you can to prevent the symptoms from coming in the first place, but keep remedies on hand for when they do flare up. If you take the measures to do this, you will quickly find that your quality of life improves drastically.

Chapter 7 –
Doctor Days: What You Should Know When Selecting The Right Doctor for You

If you have had acid reflux for any length of time, you are well aware of how many ways it can affect your life. From lack of sleep to heart and chest pain to a sore throat, it seems that your entire body is taken over by the illness.

While you can largely diagnose this disease yourself, you have also learned that there are many doctors who have misdiagnosed the symptoms due to there being many other potential reasons for you feeling the way that you do. This can make it frustrating to choose which doctor is the right medical professional for you, as you want to know for sure you are being taken care of in every way possible.

As with every other part of the medical field, there are also doctors who specialize in acid reflux and the digestive system.

Although you can't put a price on your health, you also can't help but wonder if a specialist is really necessary. The medical field is so expensive to be in, and when you start adding on medications and doctor appointments, tests and samples, and all the other things that go along with specialized treatment, it's going to get very expensive, very fast.

While there are these specialists in the field, there really are excellent options you can choose who aren't specialists. Many family doctors are able to diagnose and treat acid reflex without referring you to a specialist, especially if you already know what symptoms to watch for and what you are experiencing.

So how do you choose the right doctor for you?

If you don't already have a family doctor or a doctor that you normally see, you can shop around. Make appointments to speak with the physician and ask them questions. Many doctors are becoming more in favor of the natural lifestyle, but if you find a doctor that insists you use medication only, be willing to look around to find a doctor that is well–versed in nutrition.

Though medical schools teaches many incredible things, it is amazing how many doctors aren't given nutrition courses throughout their training, so they aren't able to point you in the right direction when it comes to natural prevention of acid reflux.

As you visit different kinds of doctors, ask which other medical professionals the doctor might recommend for other aspects of the disease you are facing – for example, ask if there is a doctor who specializes in sleep aids or natural remedies to help with sleeping problems.

The biggest mistake people make when they are choosing a medical professional to help with their acid reflux is that they refuse to ask questions.

Your doctor is a medical professional, and as such he is going to know a lot more about medical situations and answers than you are. At the same time, doctors are limited to the fields they are in, and may not have all the answers you are looking for.

If this is the case, don't be afraid to ask for another physician who is in that other field. When it comes to your health, you are never wrong to ask for more information.

Chapter 8 –
Breaking the Bad: How to Stop Doing Things to Aggravate Your Symptoms and Start Doing Things That Help

Up until this point, we have been looking at many of the dietary things you can do to help your acid reflux symptoms. It's incredibly important that you know what you can and can't eat, and why it matters, but that's not the only thing you can do to help with your acid reflux symptoms.

It seems that all too many people get so wrapped up in the dietary aspect of their acid reflux, they tend to ignore the other things they could be doing in their lives that will keep the symptoms down. In this chapter, I am going to show you the physical changes you can make to your lifestyle that will help rid you of the harmful effects of this disease.

Again, you have room to find what works for you – everyone is different, and things that work for others may not work for you, or you may find that you can tolerate and handle things others can't.

Eat smaller portions of food at a moderate pace throughout the day.

Part of the problem with acid reflux comes with how fast you eat and how much you eat. When you eat, your stomach becomes full of the food you have enjoyed until digestion moves it into the intestines. If you eat too much or too quickly, the stomach doesn't have time to process all the food before more is put on top.

This is going to lead to the stomach being distended, which will make it more likely for your sphincter at the top of your stomach to open (if it is able to close at all.)

By choosing smaller meals throughout the day, you're going to give your stomach enough time to digest and prepare for the next meal before you eat again.

Stop eating before you feel like you are entirely full.

It takes roughly 20 minutes after a meal for you to feel entirely full. This can make it difficult for you to know exactly how much you are eating, and can easily overfill your stomach.

Make a habit of stopping before you feel entirely full, and give yourself a few minutes to adjust. You'll be surprised at how much fuller you feel a few minutes after a meal than you did when you were actually eating.

Stop eating at least an hour before you lie down.

When you lie down, your stomach and esophagus are horizontal. This is going to make it far easier for your sphincter to open and for stomach acid to creep up into your esophagus – especially when you have food pushing against the top of your stomach.

When you give yourself time before you lay down, your stomach has a chance to digest the food properly, giving you greater comfort when you do lie down.

Some people find that they need to stop eating as much as two or three hours before lying down. Listen to your body and find what works best for you.

Elevate the head of your bed.

You must elevate the head of your bed itself. It's not enough to add more pillows, because lying in that position is going to put more stress and pressure on your stomach. Instead, place blocks beneath the legs at the head of your bed, so when you lie down your entire body is flat, but your head is elevated above your stomach area.

Try taking naps in a chair rather than lying down.

If you are someone who enjoys taking a nap, trying sitting in a chair to do so instead of lying down. Again, you want to keep your esophagus above your stomach without putting pressure over your stomach. By napping in a seated position, you are able to accomplish this quite well.

Wear loose fitting clothing and accessories.

Tight clothing and belts will only put more pressure on your stomach, which is going to force the stomach acid upward. Wear loose fitting clothes and avoid wearing a belt whenever possible.

Any time you can relieve rather than put pressure on your stomach, you're going to find that your symptoms of acid reflux diminish or go away completely.

If you drink or smoke, stop both.

You already known that alcohol can aggravate the symptoms of acid reflux, but smoking is also a culprit. Smoking creates more stomach acid, which is the very thing you don't want when you are dealing with the symptoms of reflux.

And, as with any other healthy lifestyle, exercise has been shown to decrease the symptoms those who are suffering from reflux feel.

Exercise alone may not be enough to alleviate your symptoms, but it's certainly going to help your body in a variety of ways. If you are overweight, exercise will help you slim down, exercise has been proven to help with digestion, and exercise will keep your body functioning properly.

In addition to doing the other things mentioned above, make an effort to include exercise into your routine three to four times per week.

Combine these things with the right diet, and you'll see your acid reflux symptoms disappear in no time!

Chapter 9 –
Acid Reflux Recipes

You've come a long way since the beginning of this book, and you have learned many things about acid reflux. But as you have seen, living the lifestyle is only part of the battle. Not only do you have to pay attention to how you eat and when you eat it, but you also need to be paying attention to what you eat.

In this final chapter, I am going to give you a variety of recipes to get you started with your new diet. Follow each of these recipes as they are written, but also pay attention to the foods that are used in these recipes and apply them to other recipes you make. When you get good at cooking for acid reflux symptoms, you will be surprised at how many things you really can eat.

Just remember to take appropriate portion sizes, to eat your meal at a moderate pace, and to eat at least ½ hour before you lie down. Use each of the preventative care techniques that you can, and you'll see those symptoms disappear in no time.

Remember to always opt for the lean meat and low fat choices with each ingredient.

Delectable Chicken Salad – Serves 2

h*What you will need:*

4 cups water

½ cup white wine

4 stalks celery

2 boneless skinless chicken breasts

4 tablespoons mayonnaise

¼ teaspoon salt

Directions:

Pour the water and the wine in a pot on the stove, and turn the stove onto medium heat. Cut the chicken into bite sized pieces and add this to the wine water mixture.

Allow the chicken to cook thoroughly on the stove, and once it has cooked through, remove from heat. Transfer to the fridge to cool for an hour.

As the chicken cools, slice the celery and combine the salt and mayo. Fold in the chicken when the time comes, then place the entire salad in the fridge to cool for another 20 minutes. Enjoy.

Best Ever Broccoli Cheese Soup – Serves 4

What you will need:

2 pounds broccoli

4 cups water

2 tsp extra virgin olive oil

½ medium white onion

2 cups skim milk

½ tsp salt

1 bag shredded cheddar cheese

4 tablespoons all purpose flour

Directions:

Start with mincing the onion into as small of pieces as you can, then cut the tops of the broccoli and shave the tough outer layer off the stems. Mince these as well once you have peeled them.

Place the broccoli in the pot of water on the stove turned onto medium high heat. Allow the broccoli to cook for 45 minutes, as this is going to make it far less likely to trigger any acid reflux symptoms.

Once the broccoli is tender, use your stick blender to puree.

Meanwhile, mince the onion into as small of pieces as you can and add to another pan on the stove. Add the olive oil and turn onto medium heat, then cook the onions until they become translucent. Add the flour and the salt, then transfer to the pot with the broccoli. Add the milk, then use your stick blender once more to puree all the ingredients.

Begin adding the cheese into the pot a little at a time, allowing each amount to melt before adding more. Reduce heat and allow to simmer for 20 minutes, and your soup is ready to enjoy.

Now That's Stroganoff – Serves 3–4

What you will need:

3 tablespoons flour

½ teaspoons pepper

2 teaspoons canola oil

1 pound flank steak

1 pound sliced mushrooms

2 tablespoons lemon juice

2 tablespoons Worcestershire sauce

¼ cup reduced fat sour cream

½ cup skim milk

1 ½ tablespoons basil

2 cups beef stock

1 teaspoon salt

1 cup nonfat sour cream

1 package egg noodles

4 cups water

Directions:

Begin by cooking the pasta in the water with the salt according to the packaging directions. As the pasta cooks, slice the flank steak into bite sized pieces and put in a pan over medium heat on the stove.

As the steak cooks, combine the remaining ingredients (except for the mushrooms) in a large bowl and set aside.

When the steak is nearly done, add the onions to the mix. Once the steak has finished cooking, add the sauce you have made. Bring the sauce to a simmer then turn down the heat and allow to simmer as the pasta finishes cooking.

Drain the pasta, then serve with the sauce over the top.

Meatball Delight – Serves 4

What you will need:

1 pound fresh beef

2 ounces fresh bread crumbs

1 teaspoon oregano

1 teaspoon basil

1 teaspoon rosemary

47

1 teaspoon thyme

½ teaspoon salt

Black pepper to taste

Cooking spray

Directions:

Preheat your oven to 400 degrees F. and spray a baking sheet with the no stick spray.

In another dish, combine all the spices and set aside. Wash your hands and combine the meat with the bread crumbs, then add the spices to the mix. Blend well.

Form into balls and line on the baking sheet. There should be around 24 small meatballs.

Cook for 10 – 15 minutes until each of the meatballs are cooked through, and serve.

Conclusion

There you have it, everything you need to know about the Acid Reflux diet, and what you can do to alleviate the symptoms you are experiencing today. I hope this book is able to give you the inspiration you need to stop the symptoms of your reflux and give you your life back.

There are so many misunderstandings about acid reflux, which makes it difficult for you to be able to know what to do to alleviate your symptoms. One person means well with the advice they offer, but another well–meaning person says the opposite. Both people wish only to help, but you are the one who has to deal with the consequences.

When it comes to the world of acid reflux, it can be easy to slip into living with dread. You never know what is going to set off your symptoms, and you never know how long they are going to last when they do start happening.

Now you know that it doesn't have to be this way. With these recipes and this new lifestyle, you know exactly what you need to do to avoid the pain and symptoms that arise with this disease. Perhaps you will be able to use this lifestyle to keep from experiencing any other symptoms in your life again.

It isn't clear whether you will be able to cure your symptoms completely, but what we do know is that you will be able to control them and keep them from happening to you severely. This the lifestyle outlined in this book, you're going to get everything you need to change the symptoms you have.

It doesn't matter how long you have been struggling with the disease, you are going to find what you need to change your symptoms for good. There's no end to the ways you can make your life more comfortable.

Think of tomorrow, and how much better you're going to feel. Think of next week, and how you'll feel even better then. Think of the week after, then the week after that. When you are living a lifestyle that promotes health, you're going to find that your symptoms simply disappear.

You are going to fall in love with the recipes, the rules, and the lifestyle that's going to offer you all the comfort you have been missing. There really is a way you can live happy and healthy, and with this new lifestyle, you can almost forget that you have acid reflux.

You can make a difference, it's just a matter of making one right choice at a time. Starting right now, you can make those choices that matter.

Good luck – now get out there and live like you mean it!